10-Minutes Flexibility Guide For Senior Over 60

A Beginner's Guide To Yoga Poses, Breathing Techniques, Building Strength, Inner Balance, Flexibility And Mindful Relaxation

Jack Simmons

Table of Contents

CHAPTER ONE

Introduction

Yoga is an ancient practice that originated in India thousands of years ago. It is a holistic discipline that combines physical postures, breath control, meditation, and ethical principles to promote physical, mental, and spiritual well-being.

The word "yoga" comes from the Sanskrit term "yuj," which means to unite or join. It reflects the idea of bringing harmony and balance to various aspects of an individual's being, including the body, mind, and spirit. Yoga is often seen as a means of achieving union between the individual self (jivatman) and the universal consciousness (Brahman).

Yoga encompasses a wide range of practices, but the most commonly known aspect of yoga in the Western world is Hatha yoga, which focuses on physical postures (asanas) and breath control (pranayama). Hatha yoga aims to balance and strengthen the body, increase flexibility, and improve overall health.

Beyond the physical aspect, yoga also involves mindfulness and meditation practices. By quieting the mind and focusing inward, practitioners aim to achieve a state of deep relaxation, self-awareness, and inner peace. Yoga is not limited to any specific religious or spiritual tradition, and it can be practiced by people of all backgrounds and belief systems.

The benefits of practicing yoga are numerous. It can help reduce stress, improve concentration and mental clarity, increase flexibility and strength, enhance overall fitness, promote emotional well-being, and cultivate a sense of inner calm and balance.

Yoga is typically taught in a group setting, led by a qualified instructor, but it can also be practiced individually. There are various styles and approaches to yoga, ranging from gentle and meditative to vigorous and dynamic. It is important to choose a style that suits your needs and physical abilities.

Whether you are looking for physical fitness, stress relief, spiritual growth, or a combination of these, yoga offers a versatile and accessible pathway to enhance your well-being and lead a more balanced and fulfilling life.

Benefits of Yoga Practice

Yoga practice emphasizes the mind-body connection, recognizing the intimate relationship between our mental and physical states. By engaging in yoga, individuals can develop a deeper understanding of this connection and experience several benefits:

Physical well-being: Yoga postures (asanas) promote strength, flexibility, and balance. Regular practice can improve posture, increase body awareness, and enhance overall physical fitness. It can also help relieve chronic pain, improve cardiovascular health, boost immune function, and promote better sleep.

Mental and emotional well-being: Yoga incorporates breath control (pranayama) and mindfulness practices, which can help calm the mind, reduce stress, and promote relaxation. Through focused breathing and meditation, individuals can cultivate a greater sense of mental clarity, emotional stability, and inner peace. Yoga has been shown to decrease symptoms of anxiety, depression, and other mental health conditions.

Stress reduction: The practice of yoga activates the body's relaxation response, which counteracts the effects of stress and promotes a sense of calm. It can help regulate the stress hormone cortisol and lower blood pressure, thereby reducing the negative impact of chronic stress on both the mind and body.

Increased self-awareness: Yoga encourages individuals to be present in the moment and develop a heightened sense of self-awareness. Through mindful movement and introspection, practitioners become more attuned to their physical sensations, thoughts, and emotions. This increased self-awareness can lead to a better understanding of one's own needs, strengths, and limitations.

Enhanced concentration and focus: Yoga practice requires concentration and attention to the body and breath. Regular practice can improve mental clarity, enhance cognitive function, and sharpen focus and attention. This can be beneficial in various aspects of life, such as work, study, and daily activities.

Emotional resilience: Yoga practice can help individuals develop emotional resilience and coping mechanisms to deal with life's challenges. By cultivating mindfulness and observing their thoughts and emotions without judgment, practitioners learn to respond to difficult situations with greater equanimity and emotional stability.

Spiritual growth: While yoga is not inherently religious, it offers a pathway for spiritual exploration and growth.

Getting Started with Yoga

Getting started with yoga involves finding a suitable yoga style that aligns with your goals and preferences, as well as gathering the essential yoga equipment. Here's a guide to help you:

Finding a Suitable Yoga Style:

Hatha Yoga: A gentle and slower-paced style that focuses on basic poses and breath control. Suitable for beginners.

Vinyasa Yoga: A dynamic style that links movement with breath, flowing through sequences of poses. Provides a good workout.

Ashtanga Yoga: A vigorous and structured style that follows a specific sequence of poses. Recommended for those seeking a physically challenging practice.

Iyengar Yoga: Emphasizes alignment and uses props to support the body in poses. Suitable for individuals with injuries or physical limitations.

Bikram Yoga/Hot Yoga: Practiced in a heated room, it consists of a fixed sequence of 26 poses. Helps promote flexibility and detoxification.

Restorative Yoga: A relaxing and passive style that uses props to support the body in restful poses. Ideal for stress relief and deep relaxation.

CHAPTER TWO

Essential Yoga Equipment

Yoga Mat: Provides cushioning and grip during poses. Look for a mat that is comfortable, durable, and appropriate for your chosen yoga style.

Comfortable Clothing: Choose breathable and stretchy attire that allows for a wide range of movement. Avoid clothes that are too loose or restrictive.

Props: Depending on the style of yoga, you may need props like blocks, straps, bolsters, or blankets to support and enhance your practice. These props can assist in modifying poses and making them more accessible.

Water Bottle: Stay hydrated throughout your practice by having a water bottle nearby.

Towel: Useful for wiping away sweat or placing over the yoga mat for better grip in hot yoga classes.

Optional: Meditation cushion or bolster, yoga strap, yoga blocks, and eye pillow can enhance your practice and support comfort during seated meditation and relaxation.

Preparing for Your Yoga Practice

Setting up a dedicated yoga space and preparing for your yoga practice can enhance your overall experience and create a peaceful and conducive environment. Here are some steps to consider:

Choose a Dedicated Space:

- Find a quiet and clutter-free area in your home where you can practice yoga without distractions.

- Ideally, select a space with natural light or good lighting that can create a calm and inviting atmosphere.

- If possible, designate a specific area solely for yoga to create a sense of sacredness and separation from everyday activities.

Clear the Space:

- Remove any objects or furniture that may obstruct your movements or cause accidents during your practice.

- Declutter the area and ensure there is enough room for you to stretch and move freely.

- Consider decorating the space with calming elements such as plants, candles, or inspiring artwork to create a serene ambiance.

Gather Your Yoga Props:

- Keep your yoga mat, blocks, straps, and any other props you use nearby in your designated space.

- Arrange them in an organized manner for easy access during your practice.

- Having your props readily available will save time and allow you to seamlessly transition between poses and sequences.

Create an Atmosphere:

- Set the mood by playing soft, soothing music or nature sounds that help you relax and focus.

- Consider using essential oils or incense to create a pleasant aroma and further enhance the ambiance.

- Adjust the temperature in the room to a comfortable level, ensuring it is neither too hot nor too cold.

Prepare Yourself:

- Wear comfortable clothing that allows for a full range of movement.

- Hydrate yourself by drinking water before and after your practice.

- Consider starting your practice with a few minutes of gentle stretching or breathing exercises to warm up your body and prepare for deeper poses.

Minimize Distractions:

Silence your phone or put it on **Do Not Disturb** mode to avoid interruptions.

Let household members know that you will be practicing yoga and request some quiet time.

If needed, hang a "Do Not Disturb" sign on the door to signal that you're engaged in your practice and should not be disturbed.

Fundamental Yoga Poses

Here are the instructions for two fundamental yoga poses: Mountain Pose (Tadasana) and Downward-Facing Dog (Adho Mukha Svanasana):

Mountain Pose (Tadasana):

- Stand tall with your feet hip-width apart, toes pointing forward, and heels slightly apart.

- Distribute your weight evenly on both feet and engage your leg muscles.

- Lengthen your spine by gently lifting the crown of your head towards the ceiling and drawing your shoulder blades back and down.

- Relax your arms by your sides, with your palms facing forward.

- Soften your facial muscles, relax your jaw, and gaze forward or gently close your eyes.

- Breathe deeply and hold the pose for 30 seconds to 1 minute, focusing on grounding and finding stability.

Downward-Facing Dog (Adho Mukha Svanasana):

- Start on your hands and knees in a tabletop position, with your wrists aligned under your shoulders and knees under your hips.

- Spread your fingers wide and press firmly into your palms, tucking your toes under.

- On an exhale, lift your knees off the ground and gradually straighten your legs, coming into an inverted V-shape.

- Keep your arms straight and shoulder-width apart, and your feet hip-width apart.

- Engage your core muscles, lengthen your spine, and press your heels towards the ground.

- Allow your head and neck to relax, with your gaze directed towards your navel or between your legs.

- Hold the pose for 5 to 10 breaths, focusing on grounding through your hands and feet while lengthening your spine.

Child's Pose (Balasana):

- Start on your hands and knees in a tabletop position.

- Bring your big toes together and widen your knees, allowing your hips to sink back towards your heels.

- Slowly lower your torso down between your thighs and rest your forehead on the mat.

- Extend your arms forward, palms facing down, or you can place them alongside your body with your palms facing up.

- Relax your shoulders, release any tension in your back, and surrender into the pose.

- Breathe deeply and hold the pose for as long as feels comfortable, typically around 1 to 3 minutes.

Warrior I (Virabhadrasana I):

- Start in a standing position with your feet hip-width apart.

- Step your left foot back, turning it out at a 45-degree angle. Your right foot should be pointing forward.

- Bend your right knee, making sure it is directly above your ankle and not extending past it.

- Square your hips forward and engage your core muscles.

- Extend your arms overhead, palms facing each other, or bring your hands to your hips for support.

- Lift your chest, lengthen your spine, and gaze forward or slightly upward.

- Breathe deeply and hold the pose for 30 seconds to 1 minute.

- Repeat the same steps on the other side, stepping your right foot back.

Tree Pose (Vrikshasana):

- Start in a standing position with your feet hip-width apart and arms by your sides.

- Shift your weight onto your left foot and lift your right foot off the ground.

- Place the sole of your right foot on your left inner thigh, avoiding placing it directly on the knee joint.

- Find your balance and bring your hands together at your heart center in a prayer position.

- Engage your core muscles and lengthen your spine.

- Find a focal point in front of you to help maintain balance.

- If you're comfortable, you can extend your arms overhead, keeping your shoulders relaxed.

- Breathe deeply and hold the pose for 30 seconds to 1 minute.

- Release the pose and repeat on the other side, placing your left foot on your right inner thigh.

Corpse Pose (Savasana):

- Lie flat on your back with your legs extended and arms relaxed by your sides, palms facing up.

- Allow your feet to fall open, and your toes to naturally relax outward.

- Close your eyes and bring your attention to your breath.

- Relax your entire body, starting from your toes and working your way up to your head.

- Let go of any tension or tightness and surrender to the support of the ground.

- Stay in this pose for 5 to 10 minutes, or longer if desired, focusing on deep relaxation and inner stillness.

CHAPTER THREE

Importance of Breath Awareness

Calms the mind:

Focusing on the breath brings attention to the present moment, helping to calm and quiet the mind.

Regulates the nervous system:

Deep, slow breathing activates the parasympathetic nervous system, triggering the relaxation response and reducing stress.

Enhances energy flow:

Pranayama techniques increase the flow of prana (life force energy) in the body, promoting vitality and overall well-being.

Improves oxygenation:

Deep breathing allows for more oxygen to be taken in and distributed throughout the body, improving energy levels and overall physical functioning.

Develops body awareness:

Breath awareness helps develop a deeper connection with the body, allowing for better understanding of sensations, emotions, and overall health.

Breathing Techniques in Yoga

Breathing techniques, also known as pranayama, play a crucial role in yoga practice. They focus on conscious control of the breath to enhance physical and mental well-being. One of the fundamental breathing techniques in yoga is deep belly breathing, also called diaphragmatic breath.

Deep Belly Breathing (Diaphragmatic Breath):

- Find a comfortable seated position, either on the floor with crossed legs or on a chair with feet flat on the ground. Sit tall with a relaxed yet upright posture.

- Place one hand on your chest and the other on your belly.

- Close your eyes or maintain a soft gaze.

- Take a slow, deep inhale through your nose, allowing your belly to expand. Feel the breath filling up the lower abdomen and lower ribs, while keeping the chest relatively still.

- Exhale slowly through your nose or mouth, feeling your belly gently contract as you expel the breath.

- Continue this deep belly breathing, focusing on the rise and fall of your abdomen with each breath.

- Maintain a steady and smooth rhythm, taking slightly longer to exhale than to inhale.

- Stay with this breath for a few minutes or longer, allowing yourself to relax and find a sense of calm.

- Deep belly breathing can be practiced on its own or integrated into your yoga poses and sequences. It can be done at any time, whether during your yoga practice, meditation, or as a standalone practice to center yourself throughout the day.

Alternate Nostril Breathing (Nadi Shodhana):

- Find a comfortable seated position, either on the floor or in a chair, with an upright yet relaxed posture.
- Rest your left hand on your left knee, palm facing up.

- Bring your right hand up to your nose, with your index and middle fingers lightly resting between your eyebrows.

- Close your right nostril with your right thumb and inhale deeply through your left nostril.

- Close your left nostril with your ring finger, release your thumb from the right nostril, and exhale fully through your right nostril.

- Inhale through your right nostril, close it with your thumb, and release your ring finger from the left nostril.

- Exhale through your left nostril.

- Continue this pattern of inhaling and exhaling, alternating between the nostrils.

- Each inhale and exhale should be slow, smooth, and deep.

- Aim to keep the breaths equal in duration, focusing on the sensation of the breath as it enters and exits the nostrils.

- Practice for a few minutes, gradually extending the duration as you become more comfortable.

Breath of Fire (Kapalabhati):

- Find a comfortable seated position, ensuring your spine is upright and relaxed.

- Place your hands on your thighs or rest them in your lap.

- Take a deep inhale through your nose, filling your belly and lungs.

- Exhale forcefully and rapidly through your nose by contracting your abdominal muscles.

- The inhalation will happen passively as you release the contraction.

- The focus is on the forceful exhale, while the inhale remains natural and relaxed.

- Start with a few rounds of rapid exhalations, gradually increasing the speed.

- After each round, take a few normal breaths to recover and observe the effects.

- Aim to build up to 3 rounds of 30-50 rapid breaths, followed by a few recovery breaths in between.

Cooling Breath (Sheetali Pranayama):

- Find a comfortable seated position, maintaining an upright posture.

- Roll your tongue into a tube-like shape or curl your tongue into a "U" shape if you can.

- If you're unable to roll or curl your tongue, simply part your lips slightly.

- Inhale slowly and deeply through the rolled or open tongue, feeling the cool air entering your mouth.

- Close your mouth and exhale slowly through your nose.

- Repeat this process for several rounds, focusing on the cooling sensation of the breath.

- Take your time with each inhalation and exhalation, savoring the refreshing quality of the breath.

- Practice for a few minutes or longer, allowing yourself to feel calm and centered.

CHAPTER FOUR

Building Flexibility through Yoga

Consistent Practice: Regularly practicing yoga helps improve flexibility over time. Dedicate time to your yoga practice, gradually increasing the duration and intensity of your sessions.

Dynamic Movements: Incorporate dynamic movements such as Sun Salutations and flowing sequences that engage multiple muscle groups. These movements help warm up the body, increase blood flow, and gradually improve flexibility.

Stretching Poses: Include stretching poses that target specific areas of the body. Some poses that can help improve flexibility include:

- Forward Folds (such as Uttanasana)
- Seated Forward
- Bend (Paschimottanasana)
- Butterfly Pose (Baddha Konasana)
- Extended Triangle Pose (Utthita Trikonasana)

Holding Poses: Hold poses for an extended period, allowing the muscles to lengthen and stretch. Poses like:

- Cobra Pose (Bhujangasana)

- Pigeon Pose (Eka Pada Rajakapotasana)

- Reclining Hand-to-Big-Toe Pose (Supta Padangusthasana)

These helps improve flexibility in specific areas.

Prop Usage: Utilize props such as blocks, straps, and bolsters to support and deepen stretches. Props can help modify poses based on your current level of flexibility and gradually increase your range of motion.

Strengthening Key Muscle Groups

Core Strength: Develop core strength through poses like:

- Plank Pose (Phalakasana)

- Boat Pose (Navasana)

- Side Plank (Vasisthasana)

These poses engage the abdominal muscles, obliques, and back muscles, providing stability and strength.

Upper Body Strength: Poses like:

- Downward-Facing Dog (Adho Mukha Svanasana)

- Chaturanga Dandasana (Four-Limbed Staff Pose)

- Crow Pose (Bakasana)

These helps strengthen the arms, shoulders, and upper back. Incorporating these poses into your practice can improve upper body strength and stability.

Lower Body Strength: Poses such as:

- Warrior I (Virabhadrasana I),

- Warrior II (Virabhadrasana II)

- Chair Pose (Utkatasana)

These build strength in the legs, glutes, and hips. These poses help increase stability, endurance, and overall lower body strength.

Balance Poses: Balance poses like:

- Tree Pose (Vrikshasana)
- Eagle Pose (Garudasana)
- Warrior III (Virabhadrasana III)

These challenges and strengthen the muscles in the legs, ankles, and feet. Practicing these poses improves balance, stability, and lower body strength.

Balancing Poses for Core Strength

Some balancing poses that can help strengthen the core:

Sun Salutation (Surya Namaskar): Sun Salutation is a dynamic sequence of yoga poses that helps warm up the body, stretch and strengthen various muscle groups, and connect breath with movement. It consists of several poses performed in a flowing sequence. Here is a simplified version of Sun Salutation:

Mountain Pose (Tadasana): Stand tall with feet together or hip-width apart, palms together at your heart center.

Upward Salute (Urdhva Hastasana): Inhale, raise your arms overhead, gently arching your back and looking up.

Forward Fold (Uttanasana): Exhale, hinge at the hips, and fold forward, bringing your hands to the floor beside your feet.

Halfway Lift (Ardha Uttanasana): Inhale, lengthen your spine, bringing your fingertips to your shins or thighs, gaze forward.

Plank Pose: Exhale, step or jump back to a high plank position, with your hands under your shoulders and legs extended.

Chaturanga Dandasana: Lower down with control, bending your elbows close to your sides, keeping your body parallel to the ground.

Upward-Facing Dog (Urdhva Mukha Svanasana): Inhale, press through your hands, straighten your arms, lift your chest, and roll over your toes, keeping your legs off the ground.

Downward-Facing Dog (Adho Mukha Svanasana): Exhale, lift your hips up and back, forming an inverted V-shape, pressing your palms into the ground.

To complete the sequence, you can step or jump your feet forward between your hands, returning to Forward Fold (Uttanasana), and then rise up to Mountain Pose (Tadasana). Repeat the sequence for several rounds, synchronizing each movement with your breath.

Boat Pose (Navasana): Sit on the floor with your knees bent and feet flat on the ground. Lean back slightly, lift your feet off the ground, balancing on your sit bones. Extend your legs to a straight position, forming a "V" shape with your body. Engage your core muscles and keep your spine straight. You can hold onto the backs of your thighs or extend your arms parallel to the floor. Hold for a few breaths and gradually increase the duration as you build strength.

Warrior III (Virabhadrasana III): Start in Mountain Pose (Tadasana). Shift your weight onto your right foot and hinge forward at the hips, extending your left leg behind you. Simultaneously extend your arms forward, palms facing each other. Engage your core to maintain balance and create a straight line from your head to your left foot. Hold for several breaths, then switch sides.

Tree Pose (Vrikshasana): Begin in Mountain Pose (Tadasana). Shift your weight onto your left foot and place the sole of your right foot on your inner left thigh or calf, avoiding placing it directly on the knee joint. Find your balance and bring your hands together at your heart center. Engage your core and lengthen your spine. Hold for several breaths, then switch sides.

CHAPTER FIVE

Importance of Relaxation in Yoga

Reduces Stress: Relaxation techniques in yoga activate the parasympathetic nervous system, which helps counteract the effects of stress on the body. It promotes relaxation, lowers heart rate, and reduces levels of stress hormones like cortisol.

Enhances Mind-Body Connection: Relaxation allows you to cultivate a deeper connection between your mind and body. By consciously relaxing, you become more aware of sensations, emotions, and the present moment.

Restores Energy: Taking time to relax rejuvenates the body and mind, replenishing energy levels. It helps alleviate fatigue and improves overall vitality.

Supports Healing and Recovery: Relaxation promotes the body's natural healing processes and helps in recovery from physical exertion, injuries, or illness. It supports better sleep, reduces muscle tension, and aids in pain management.

Yoga Nidra (Yogic Sleep)

Preparation: Find a comfortable spot where you can lie down without any distractions. Use a bolster, blanket, or any props that support your body's comfort. Cover yourself with a light blanket to stay warm.

Intention Setting: Before beginning Yoga Nidra, set an intention or sankalpa. It can be a positive affirmation or a personal goal you want to manifest. Repeat your sankalpa silently to yourself, such as "I am calm and peaceful" or "I am filled with love and compassion."

Guided Instructions: Follow a guided Yoga Nidra recording or the instructions of a qualified instructor. The guide will lead you through various stages of relaxation, body awareness, breath awareness, visualization, and deepening relaxation.

Deep Relaxation: During Yoga Nidra, you enter a state of deep relaxation where your body and mind experience profound rest. It is a practice of surrendering, letting go, and allowing yourself to be fully present in the moment.

Witnessing Awareness: In Yoga Nidra, you cultivate the practice of witnessing awareness. You observe your thoughts, emotions, and sensations without judgment or attachment. You remain aware of the experiences that arise without getting caught up in them.

Yoga for Stress Relief

Gentle and Restorative Yoga: Choose gentle and restorative yoga styles that focus on slow, deliberate movements, deep breathing, and relaxation. These styles help calm the nervous system and reduce stress. Examples include Yin

Yoga, Restorative Yoga, and Hatha Yoga.

Mindfulness and Meditation: Incorporate mindfulness and meditation practices into your yoga routine. This helps cultivate present-moment awareness, reduce mental chatter, and promote a sense of calm. Mindful breathing exercises and guided meditations can be beneficial for stress relief.

Breathing Techniques: Explore different pranayama (breathing) techniques to help regulate and calm the breath, which in turn can help calm the mind and reduce stress. Deep belly breathing, alternate nostril breathing, and extended exhale breathing are effective techniques for stress relief.

Stress-Relieving Poses: Include poses that target areas prone to holding tension, such as the neck, shoulders, and hips. Gentle stretches, forward folds, and twists can help release physical and mental stress.

- Child's Pose (Balasana)
- Legs-Up-The-Wall Pose (Viparita Karani)

- Supine Spinal Twist (Supta Matsyendrasana)

These are examples of poses that can promote relaxation.

Prenatal Yoga

Gentle and Modified Poses: Practice gentle yoga poses that are modified to accommodate the changes in the body during pregnancy. Focus on poses that promote strength, flexibility, and relaxation, while avoiding excessive pressure on the abdomen. Prenatal yoga classes specifically tailored for pregnant women are ideal.

Pelvic Floor Exercises: Incorporate exercises to strengthen the pelvic floor muscles, which support the uterus, bladder, and bowel. Kegels and modified versions of poses like Bridge Pose (Setu Bandha Sarvangasana) can be beneficial.

Breath Awareness: Utilize breathing techniques like diaphragmatic breathing and modified pranayama to support relaxation and enhance breath awareness, which can be helpful during labor and childbirth.

Postnatal Yoga

Gentle and Restorative Practices: Begin with gentle and restorative yoga practices to aid in postpartum recovery. Focus on gentle stretches, relaxation, and reconnecting with the body. Pelvic floor exercises and core-strengthening poses can be gradually introduced as healing progresses.

Mindful Movement: Pay attention to your body's needs and limitations postpartum. Modify poses as necessary and practice mindfulness during movement to ensure proper healing and prevent overexertion.

Bonding with Baby: Incorporate poses and practices that allow for bonding with your baby, such as baby-friendly poses and gentle movements that involve interaction and closeness.

When practicing yoga during pregnancy or after giving birth, it's crucial to consult with a qualified prenatal/postnatal yoga instructor who can guide you through safe and appropriate modifications for your specific needs.

CHAPTER SIX

Chair Yoga for Limited Mobility

Seated Poses: Modify traditional yoga poses to be performed while seated on a chair. This allows individuals with limited mobility to access the benefits of yoga. Seated forward folds, twists, gentle stretches, and upper body movements can be incorporated.

Joint Mobility and Range of Motion: Focus on gentle movements that promote joint mobility and increase range of motion. Ankle and wrist rotations, shoulder rolls, and neck stretches can help improve flexibility and reduce stiffness.

Breathing and Meditation: Emphasize breath awareness and incorporate meditation techniques that can be practiced comfortably while seated. Deep belly breathing and guided visualizations can help promote relaxation and reduce stress.

Mind-Body Connection: Encourage participants to cultivate mindfulness and body awareness during chair yoga practice. This involves paying attention to sensations, breath, and thoughts without judgment.

Yoga for Seniors

Gentle and Accessible Poses: Choose poses that are gentle, accessible, and adaptable to the needs and abilities of seniors. Focus on improving strength, balance, flexibility, and stability. Standing poses, seated poses, gentle flows, and supported inversions can be included.

Chair Modifications: Utilize chairs or other props to provide stability and support during poses. This can help seniors with balance issues or limited mobility to practice yoga safely.

Fall Prevention and Balance: Incorporate poses and exercises that improve balance and reduce the risk of falls. One-legged balance poses, modified tree pose, and simple standing balance exercises can be beneficial.

Breathwork and Relaxation: Integrate breathwork techniques, such as diaphragmatic breathing and alternate nostril breathing, to promote relaxation and stress reduction. Include guided relaxation or Yoga Nidra practices to facilitate deep rest and rejuvenation.

Yoga for Children and Teens

Playful and Engaging Approach: Make yoga sessions fun, interactive, and age-appropriate to keep children and teens engaged. Incorporate storytelling, games, music, and creative visualization to make the practice enjoyable.

Mindful Movement and Breath: Introduce basic yoga poses, emphasizing mindful movement and breath awareness. Teach children and teens to connect with their bodies and breath, promoting self-awareness and emotional regulation.

Partner Poses and Group Activities: Encourage partner poses and group activities to foster cooperation, trust, and teamwork. This allows children and teens to develop social skills while exploring yoga postures together.

Mindfulness and Relaxation: Introduce mindfulness exercises and relaxation techniques tailored to the age group. Guided visualizations, body scans, and mindful breathing can help children and teens manage stress, improve focus, and enhance overall well-being.

When working with individuals with specific needs or age groups, it's beneficial to consult with specialized yoga instructors who have experience in chair yoga, senior yoga, or yoga for children and teens. They can provide appropriate modifications, guidance, and support to ensure a safe and enjoyable practice for everyone involved.

The frequency of your yoga practice

The frequency of your yoga practice depends on your personal schedule and goals. Ideally, aim for at least 2-3 sessions per week to maintain consistency and experience the benefits of yoga. As you progress and feel more comfortable, you can gradually increase the frequency and duration of your practice. However, even a short daily practice of 10-15 minutes can be beneficial.

Yoga Clothing

Regarding what to wear for yoga, choose clothing that allows for ease of movement and is comfortable. Opt for breathable, stretchy fabrics that allow your body to move freely without restriction. Yoga leggings, shorts, or sweatpants, paired with a comfortable top or a fitted sports bra, are common choices. Avoid overly loose or baggy clothing that may hinder your movement or get in the way during poses. Additionally, consider wearing layers to adjust for temperature fluctuations during your practice.

Remember, the most important aspect of your yoga practice is your mindset and willingness to show up on the mat. It's not about how flexible or advanced you are, but rather about your commitment to self-care, self-discovery, and the journey of personal growth that yoga offers. Embrace where you are in your practice and enjoy the process of deepening your mind-body connection through yoga.

Conclusion

The journey of yoga is an ongoing process of self-discovery, self-care, and personal growth. It's a practice that extends beyond the physical postures and encompasses the integration of mind, body, and spirit.

Ultimately, yoga is a personal journey that unfolds uniquely for each individual. Embrace the process, stay committed, and allow yourself to experience the physical, mental, and spiritual benefits that yoga has to offer. With an open heart and a willingness to explore, you'll discover the profound and transformative effects of yoga in your life.

THE END